Lighten Up America

3/15/17

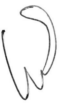

LIGHTEN UP AMERICA

Odds and Not So Fat Ends of Weight Management

FROM the *FAMILY PRACTICE DIARIES BOOK 1*

Lisa Clark MD, Family Medicine

Edited by P. J. Heslin

iUniverse, Inc.
Bloomington

LIGHTEN UP AMERICA
ODDS AND NOT SO FAT ENDS OF WEIGHT MANAGEMENT

Copyright © 2013 Lisa Clark MD, Family Medicine.

All rights reserved. No part of this book may be used or reproduced by any means, graphic, electronic, or mechanical, including photocopying, recording, taping or by any information storage retrieval system without the written permission of the publisher except in the case of brief quotations embodied in critical articles and reviews.

You should not undertake any diet/exercise regimen recommended in this book before consulting your personal physician. Neither the author nor the publisher shall be responsible or liable for any loss or damage allegedly arising as a consequence of your use or application of any information or suggestions contained in this book.

iUniverse books may be ordered through booksellers or by contacting:

iUniverse
1663 Liberty Drive
Bloomington, IN 47403
www.iuniverse.com
1-800-Authors (1-800-288-4677)

Because of the dynamic nature of the Internet, any web addresses or links contained in this book may have changed since publication and may no longer be valid. The views expressed in this work are solely those of the author and do not necessarily reflect the views of the publisher, and the publisher hereby disclaims any responsibility for them.

Any people depicted in stock imagery provided by Thinkstock are models, and such images are being used for illustrative purposes only.

Certain stock imagery © Thinkstock.

ISBN: 978-1-4620-5717-7 (sc)
ISBN: 978-1-4620-5718-4 (hc)
ISBN: 978-1-4620-5719-1 (e)

Library of Congress Control Number: 2013908258

Printed in the United States of America.

iUniverse rev. date: 6/6/2013

Contents

Acknowledgments................vii

Introduction.....................xi

PART ONE
EDUCATION IS THE KEY...............1

Chapter 1   No Magic Required............3

Chapter 2   The Scary Truth about Obesity........15

Chapter 3   Could It Be My Thyroid? I'm Really Hoping!.....21

Chapter 4   Exercise with a Purpose............27

PART TWO
AGE AND WEIGHT................37

Chapter 5   Infants, Kids, and Weight Management.......39

Chapter 6   Teens and Weight Management........49

Chapter 7   The Postpartum Weight Struggle........53

Chapter 8   Menopause and Weight Management 61

Chapter 9   Men and Weight Management 67

PART THREE
MOTIVATE THYSELF 75

Chapter 10 Supplements and Diet Aids 77

Chapter 11 Odds and Not-So-Fat Ends 79

Chapter 12 A Patient Success Story 81

It's A Wrap 83

About the Author 85

Notes 87

Acknowledgments

I need to mention several people who helped make this book possible.

First, I want to thank my mom, who always stressed that I was capable of anything I set my mind to. She has been a constant in my life, whether I needed help or just needed to laugh. She helped with childcare so I could finish my residency and open my practice, and today she continues to be a friend, super-mom, and super-grandma! When I was five, my parents adopted my sister and three brothers. I watched as my mom juggled family and work while still making time to exercise. Her example demonstrated to us that exercise is important. Today she continues to play tennis, travel, and keep very active, and I am proud of all she has accomplished.

My Bobchee and Geejaw (Polish for "Grandma" and "Grandpa") taught me the importance of a good work ethic. They kept constantly in motion, never sitting still, and I believe that was the reason they lived so many quality years. They are the example to which I will refer when talking about lifestyles two generations ago. They have been and still are an inspiration to me in all I do.

I need to thank my kids, Adam and Ava, who have put up with Mom running her practice and constantly trying to fit in a workout, even if it meant that I stuffed Adam into a stroller he had slightly outgrown so I could get in a run. I want to thank my kids for their sunny outlook on life and their sense of humor, which I could not do without. Adam and Ava are often the jesters, but sometimes the audience!

My husband, Michael, continued to believe that I would finish this book, even though, it has been several years in the creative phase (okay, the dormant phase). With his encouragement and support, I could have time for myself to run, write, work, and even train for my first marathon.

My sisters, Reanne, Mindy, and Nikki, have shared diet stories and endless hours of laughter with me, and they have always believed in me. Sisters are the best source of diet information—not always the best source of advice, but the best role models for learning to laugh at yourself and to accept that you may never have that figure of a 12-year-old boy that you have always wanted.

My big brother, P. J., helped edit this book and helped me realize my goal of completing a marathon at the age of forty-three. An experienced marathoner, he ran beside me for 5 hours and 26 minutes as I completed something I had always wanted to do. I am now training for my third marathon. He collaborated with me, especially on the chapter on exercise, and he offered valuable guidance on the chapter for men. He has completed an ultramarathon and several triathlons and marathons, and he continues to defy the properties of cartilage. (I think he was born with knee and hip replacements.) He may be the funniest guy I know, and I am constantly entertained by his sense of humor and love for life.

My nurse, Keta, has been with me longer than any doctor could expect a nurse to hang around. Her sense of humor and her steadfast loyalty are invaluable to my practice. She keeps her smile even after ten patients in a row try to kill her with their eyes for asking them to step on the scale, as if it were her fault that they were overweight and depressed. She is not only the most loyal employee, but also has become my best friend. We have shared endless hours of patient care—sometimes funny, sometimes stressful. She keeps me straight and tries to keep me focused. She has even colored my hair when the gray started to show. She is truly my gal Friday!

Also, I would like to mention my dad, who was diagnosed with type 2 diabetes mellitus and was able to control it with diet and exercise. Many diagnosed patients figure that if they take the pill, they can eat whatever they want. A onetime marathoner himself, Dad also encouraged me to reach my dream of completing a marathon. I thought about him often while training for my first marathon and during the marathon, and he is still an inspiration to me in my running.

Lastly and *most importantly, I want to acknowledge my patients,* whom I have spent many hours trying to help with weight management. I have learned more from them than they have from me. I continue to be inspired and impressed at the hard work that goes into a person bettering themselves. I thank all who have trusted me as a physician and I am grateful to have had the opportunity to serve as a family-practice doctor. My patients and I have shared laughter, tears, frustration, success, and all the other emotions in between.

Introduction

This book was originally written to aid my patients with weight management. After working in clinical medicine for fourteen years, and spending thousands of hours discussing weight loss with my patients, I knew that a handbook with the important points I discussed every day could help people looking for advice. Such answers are not always available from personal trainers or in diet books.

The book is divided into three sections. Part One, "Education Is the Key," considers the following question: What is the secret to losing weight and really maintaining a comfortable, healthy body weight? This section will address how to understand calories. My hope is that it will help you learn how to balance calories *in* versus calories *out* (the real answer to weight loss). In addition, this section focuses on the dangers of obesity and other health problems associated with obesity, as well as answering the question "Could it be my thyroid?"

Part Two, "Age and Weight," addresses the life stages of battling weight, from infancy to adulthood. You will learn the commonsense information that can help you attain a healthy weight—not as part of a crash diet, but as part of a healthy lifestyle. These chapters, designed for women, take into account the special considerations of children, teenagers, postpartum women, and postmenopausal women—though men can certainly find them helpful as well. I've also developed a chapter just for men. Included is just enough information so the readers with ADD (attention deficit disorder) can get through it before losing interest.

Finally, Part Three, "Motivate Thyself," gives tips and advice on developing discipline and making healthy choices.

My goal is to educate patients on achieving and maintaining an ideal body weight while adding some humor to the subject. I have not created any special fad; you won't see this as the featured diet of the month on the cover of *Redbook*, or any other grocery store magazine. I have no special foods or shakes to sell—in fact, I have nothing to sell other than my experience with the subject. In North America, childhood obesity is on the rise, and type 2 diabetes cases are rapidly increasing as well. In light of the scary statistics, I hope to prevent the long-term complications that can result from being overweight.

As you read on, I hope you will find many helpful ideas. If you have children, I hope you can teach our next generation the importance of exercising, eating well, and managing food intake by setting great examples. With the help of the ideas and discussion presented here, you will be in charge of maintaining a healthy body weight and feeling comfortable in your own skin.

As a family doctor, I get the privilege of becoming familiar with the entire family dynamic. It allows me a wonderful insight into how families think about weight and exercise. I often see that when I work with one part of that system, the rest follows suit, and it is rewarding to see evidence of those healthy lifestyle changes.

You've taken a great first step in picking up this book! And if you decide you don't want to read it, regift it to a fat friend or family member. They will be forever grateful.

My goal has always been to teach and inform, so you can teach and inform yourself.

Let's come together as a nation to evolve into the next era and find an answer to "forget the fat"!

Part One
EDUCATION IS THE KEY

Chapter 1

No Magic Required

Is there a magic pill or magic diet that could help you lose twenty pounds in two weeks and look sexy for life? If there were, you wouldn't be reading this. You would not see a new diet of the month on the cover of every magazine in the grocery store.

Losing weight, and keeping it off, requires no magic. In this chapter, you will find the information you need to lose weight and maintain.

With that in mind, remember the first line from the book *The Road Less Traveled*: life is difficult! Well guess what? LOSING WEIGHT IS DIFFICULT. Even more difficult is keeping off the weight you lose.

If you are reading this book, you've probably already tried a lot of diets.

The most important step you can take toward your weight-loss goals is to educate yourself about calories. If you want to lose weight, you have to keep track of calories, find out exactly what your body requires to lose weight, and then maintain the weight you want. In other words, how many calories can you eat in a day and still lose weight? Once you've reached your desired weight, you'll also need to determine how many calories you can eat in a day while still maintaining the weight you desire.

If you are going to proceed with the book and my ideas about managing weight, you are going to have to understand the importance of tracking calories. It has to be done on a daily basis—and you have to be accurate.

My experience has been that patients who are successful at long-term weight management are those who keep *honest* food journals. Yes, snacks count, and so do those mini chocolate bars you have in your office drawer. Only about 10 percent of all patients I see for weight management keep food journals.

Thanks to technology and the web, calorie tracking is easier. When I first started practicing medicine, you would have had to buy a book in which to look up the number of calories in your food. Now, so many apps track calories; you simply enter what you have eaten, and the caloric content pops up. If you don't have a smart phone, you can find many websites that will do similar work for you. Those of you still living in Bedrock (Fred Flintstone's hometown) can still go to the bookstore and buy a book of calorie counts.

If you learn how to apply the basic principle of calories in and calories out, you can understand how your body stores calories and then turns them to fat. This means learning the caloric content of what you are eating, and what your body requires for losing and then maintaining weight. Although the idea seems easy enough to understand, the execution is difficult, which is why this information is so important.

A food journal will help you track your calories. Food journals are where most of my patients struggle. They may keep track of caloric intake for a day or a week, but very few will do this over the period of a month. A month is the minimum amount of time needed to provide an accurate idea of the amount of fuel going in. I have had patients bring me in a few things written down on a cocktail napkin. Really? The day before your visit, you scratched down a few things on a cocktail napkin while having a margarita after a long day at work? It's funny, but not helping either of us figure out how many calories your body needs to lose weight.

If you are familiar with how a business profits (or loses money), you can think of the calorie journal as a profit and loss statement. Money comes in, and money comes out. If you spend more than you make, you will go bankrupt. In the case of calories, if you eat more than you burn, you will gain weight and get fat. (I can use the word *fat* because I was fat at one point: five-foot-five and 190 pounds. Yikes.)

You can't possibly be successful at budgeting your money *or* losing weight if you don't watch the numbers. If you are not familiar with profit and loss, think of your calorie journal as your debit card or checkbook. If you don't keep track of your remaining balance, your card may get declined, or your check might bounce. The other analogy I like to use with patients is driving without a speedometer. If you don't have one, or it's broken, you will undoubtedly speed. Keeping an eye on the numbers is just as important in weight loss. I actually did drive without a speedometer for a few months, and its true you will drive too fast and get a ticket.

If you are serious about weight management, then this is your number-one priority: educate yourself and become familiar with caloric needs in order to make permanent healthy changes in your life. Remember, we all have different requirements, so you can't follow what your friend, husband, wife, or sister is consuming. Your plan needs to be designed for you.

Know about Calories

To start your food journal, you'll need a written record of your daily intake of food and calories. **Do not guess!** And be honest—don't make stuff up and bring it to your doctor. You are only lying to yourself.

You can use a traditional paper notebook, a computer-based journal, an online site, or an app, as mentioned earlier. Whether you have an iPhone, Android phone, or BlackBerry, you'll be able to find an app that very easily allows you to track calories.

Start by entering all the foods and beverages you take in daily, To maximize your weight management, you will also have to exercise, but don't make the mistake of telling yourself, "I exercised today, so I can eat that chocolate ice-cream sundae." No, you can't, if you are trying to lose weight. The exercise is a bonus, and a lot of trainers and apps tell you to subtract the calories burned from your day's total. But don't—keep your calories to the number you need to lose weight, and add exercise as a bonus. You will read more later about how to exercise with a purpose.

So this is the question: how many calories should you take in daily? So many trainers and books offer different answers. On average, I have found that women need no more than an average of 1,200 calories a day to lose weight, and men need about 1,600 a day. That is not a lot, but I have come up with these numbers by watching my patients, and also by monitoring my own weight and caloric intake. I found that I could not take in more than 1,200 a day, or I would remain static. That is what frustrates so many people. They may lose a few pounds before stabilizing at a certain weight, and then throw in the towel and get an ice-cream sundae. That's not going to work, as most of you have already found.

One of my favorite questions to ask in my initial or even follow-up visits with my patients who see me for weight management is, "How many calories are you taking in daily, on average?"

The answer frequently is, "Umm, let's see, well, I don't eat that much …"

So I listen as they fumble around, trying to guess what they have eaten.

"Well, I've had a lot of salads and fruits, and I'm eating healthy …"

"So you have no idea how many calories you're eating."

"You are correct, sir."

Then we laugh, and I go into my spiel about the importance of knowing your caloric intake. You need to know exactly what you are eating; if you cheat, you are wasting your own time.

It may seem that 1,200 to 1,600 calories is a low intake. It is, and in today's world, it's all too easy to consume this much in one meal. A McDonald's Quarter Pounder value meal, with fries and a soft drink, is 1,190 calories! And that's just one meal. Avoid fast foods and choose the healthier option like a wrap instead of a burger at McDonalds.

A lot of other weight information will tell you that women need 1,800 calories and men need 2,000 a day. There's no way you can lose weight taking in this many calories. How do I know? I've tried it!

Remember, too, that we are no longer churning butter on the farm with a baby on our back, plowing the fields from sunup to sundown while feeding the chickens and cows, herding the sheep, and fighting off wolves. Think about it: you've probably never seen an overweight farmer, roofer, or landscape worker. These are people who burn everything they put into their bodies, and the principle applies to you as well. Many of us are now spending our days sitting at a desk in front of a computer screen, not scavenging for nuts and fruits.

Know What You're Eating

While our grandparents and even parents may have walked six miles to school one way in the snow, we are lucky if we walk to the fridge, and if our television remotes fail, we're stranded like turtles on their backs. We do not burn the same number of calories as a society as we did a hundred or even fifty years ago. Do you ever see pictures of obese pioneers? No, because their day was consumed with activity, and their caloric input was equal to what they required. Very few type 2 diabetics could be found at that time, due to the lack of overeating. Food was not constantly at arm's reach. As we have evolved into a society where we have motorized means to transport us, and our work no longer involves much more exercise than using our fingers or thumbs to type. We are all hooked to some kind of mobile device and we have evolved into obese, sedentary, overeaters. Darwin would be confused and disappointed!

So, its time to evolve our habits and activity to meet the evolution of inactivity.

We have become a society about food. Caloric evil lurks behind every corner, providing us with excuses such as:

- It was my office mate's birthday today

- It was my turn to bring the king cake for Mardi Gras.

- A drug representative brought in doughnuts from Krispy Kreme—and the "hot and fresh" light was on! (Guess what? It's *always* on.)

My personal favorite is "It's the holidays." Yes, it is the damn holidays, but you don't have to eat like a wild boar. Or, if you are going to eat like a wild boar, how about getting a little exercise before you sit down to tear apart some unlucky turkey? Don't get me wrong. I love turkey and stuffing and gravy—sometimes all three at once. I love Christmas cookies and cake and bread. Who doesn't like fresh-baked bread? But we have to get to a point where we ask ourselves, "Am I eating because I'm hungry, or just because it tastes so good?"

You have to train your mind to ask this question: "Am I hungry?" You may be thirsty, and instead of a glass of water, you reach for food. That is why so many weight-loss books advise you to drink some ungodly amount of water a day. Instead of keeping water at your side in the Big Glug jug you got at a gas station, learn to ask yourself this important question: "Am I hungry?"

If the answer is no, step away from the food, put down the day-old doughnut, and avoid getting seconds. You will be challenged daily, hourly—when you pass the vending machine, the hot-dog cart, the ice-cream store. Get rid of the emergency *Three Musketeers* bar in your desk drawer. If there is an emergency, we will call the ambulance for you!

This is the hard part of weight management, and I am not going to lie to you and say it's easy. People have tried to find the magic answer to being thin, but guess what? There is none. I wish I had a magic answer, but I don't, and as far as I can tell, no one else does, either. There is no easy solution to managing a healthy body weight, at least not in our society today.

If our society had found a diet that worked, would magazines be offering new tricks in every issue? "Get thin by Labor Day!" "Slim down by Christmas!" "Drop pounds by Memorial Day!" "Fit into your bikini by July 4!" How many issues have you bought thinking,

This time, I'm really going to lose weight and look great before the family reunion in three months, only to lose four pounds, get stuck, get frustrated, and then give up? There is no secret, and there are no special foods you need to buy.

This book is not a diet book. Here is my secret: There is no secret. You simply have to work to become familiar with the caloric content of food. It is a pain in the ass to get started, but it will be worth it.

Those of you who have quit smoking, or tried, know it's so hard because cigarettes seem to be everywhere when you're trying to quit. Plus, the habit of smoking is intertwined with the rest of your life. You're used to smoking after a meal, while having a drink, or as a break at work. But eventually (after the initial nicotine withdrawal), you learn to not associate every activity with smoking. Similarly, we don't have to eat everything put in front of us. In fact, we can change what we put in front of us—and we can change the way we think about food.

So you start to look at the caloric intake of your favorite spaghetti sauce, along with your favorite cereal and salad dressing. We are creatures of habit; we buy the same food items, use the same products, eat the same meals. That is okay, but it's time to see just where those calories are hiding. If your favorite snack is fat-free, that doesn't mean it has no calories. How many calories are in your favorite fat-free yogurt? If it's 200 calories, these little snack items can start to add up, especially if paired with your regular meals during the day. You might say to yourself, "But I only ever eat salads." That may be true, but how many calories are in the ranch dressing you're covering it with?

The education starts here. Investigate the caloric content of your most common food items—by law, this information is on the labels—and when you eat out. Don't worry, most restaurants have the calorie content available. It's easier than ever to track your caloric intake. If you don't do this, you will never be able to manage your intake (and therefore your weight).

Over and over, I have found that those patients who understand why they have a disease or illness are much more likely to be compliant with treatment. So I often spend a few extra minutes explaining to them how their bodies have developed their particular problem, how we can fix it, what other possibilities may exist, and what to do if the initial instructions fail. This extra ten minutes leaves the patient with the feeling that they have an answer; I rarely get phone calls later regarding their visit.

> **Case Study: Bob**
>
> Bob was a forty-year-old, 350-pounds smoker with high blood pressure and high cholesterol. He came to see me because his regular doctor was out of town. His blood pressure was sky high, and he was taking his meds intermittently—and, of course, still smoking. I asked him whether he understood what hypertension, or high blood pressure was, and how smoking affected this, and how high cholesterol and obesity were intertwined with all these problems. Smoking and cholesterol had narrowed his arteries, making his heart and lungs work harder. His weight affected all his body systems, too.
>
> He knew very little, and I took some time to explain some of these problems to him—how he was at risk for a heart attack, a stroke, degenerative joint disease, and other long-term complications related to being overweight. On our next visit, he was taking his meds regularly, his blood pressure was down to normal, and he had cut back on his smoking significantly. He had also lost ten pounds, was walking, and was of course feeling better than he had in years.

The point of this story is that patients who understand how weight loss works are more likely to succeed and keep off the weight permanently. The simple answer is that to lose weight, you must put in fewer calories a day than you were burning.

Sample Food Diary

Food Eaten	Calorie Intake	Calories Burned
Half cup cereal and half cup skim milk	200 calories	
Tea w/ 1 tsp sugar and 1 tsp skim milk	20	
Apple	40	
Takeout chicken wrap	300	
Diet Coke	0	
2 pieces gum	10	
Handful of chips	50	
Pasta with sauce (small portion)	300	
Salad with dressing	150	
Plum	30	
Half power bar	100	
Total for day	1,200	
Exercise - 30 minutes slow jog		<150>
Net daily calories	1,050	

Chapter Summary

Most people have struggled with weight during their lives, or know someone who has.

- Knowledge is the key to empowering yourself to maintain a healthy, comfortable body weight.

- You must burn more calories than you take in daily to succeed in losing weight.

- No magic powders, foods, or pills will allow you to maintain a weight that is necessary for maintaining long-term health and quality of life.

Chapter 2

The Scary Truth about Obesity

If being overweight or obese and being tired of shopping in the big-and-tall section isn't enough motivation for you, let me give you a scarier version of that motivation: *comorbidity*.

Comorbidity? Yikes, that sounds like death. Yes, it is meant to sound like death! If you add obesity to any other medical condition, you will have to visit my office much more often.

Much of what I have to say about this will not be surprising, but sometimes, it helps to drive home the physical benefits of maintaining a healthy weight—they go way beyond looking good in yoga pants, and skinny jeans.

Weight affects the entire rest of your body, how it functions, and how it starts to break down. Haven't you seen those people who are twenty-eight years old and look fifty, and then those who are fifty, but look twenty-eight? How can this be explained? There's the obvious smoking and drinking that age people twice as fast, and then there is obesity. Add all three and throw in some yellow teeth you have an extremely old looking person.

Below you will find information on how obesity affects your different body systems. It doesn't yellow your teeth, as far as I know, so get them bleached after you are done reading.

Heart Disease

Most everyone is aware that those who are overweight and sedentary—couch potatoes, in other words—have an increased chance of having a heart attack or stroke. Patients who have suffered these can still be reluctant or unable to maintain a healthy weight. How many fat old people have you seen? That's right—not many because most of them have died from weight-related problems or a sedentary lifestyle. I don't mean to say that all people who have died young had unhealthy lives. We all know of someone who did all the right things, but got unlucky with breast cancer, leukemia, or something similarly tragic. That seems damn unfair when you look at someone who is eighty-five, smokes two packs a day, and is drinking alcohol by 10:00 a.m. Fear not—they can't feel great!

If you already have risk factors for coronary heart disease (heart attack), you need to take your weight seriously. Other risk factors besides weight include a family history of heart disease, high cholesterol (check this at least once by the time you are thirty, and then yearly after that), smoking, a history of high blood pressure and diabetes, and an age of more than fifty years old. Doctors assess these common risk factors when patients present with chest pain. Also, if you are at risk for heart disease (and don't forget: women will present differently than men), ask your doctor to set you up for a stress test. This involves being hooked up to an EKG while running on a treadmill while your doctor looks for any concerning changes in the EKG during exercise.

Diabetes

Another system that is often adversely affected by obesity is the endocrine system, which comprises a set of glands that affect hormone secretion. These include the thyroid gland, parathyroid glands, and pituitary gland. All are important.

Adult-onset diabetes is big problem. Every year, I diagnose many overweight, out-of-shape patients with diabetes, most of whom have a family history of the disease. The importance of exercise cannot be emphasized enough in the control and prevention of type 2 diabetes. When I ask patients how they are doing with exercise and weight control, many look sheepishly at me and say, "I know. I need to do better." I also have motivated patients who save hundreds of dollars a month on meds by controlling their blood sugar with diet and exercise.

If either of your parents have adult diabetes, don't wait until you get it. Start exercising regularly, maintain a healthy body weight, and don't eat too much crap! Now we are seeing type 2 diabetes in kids, and so our society is starting to take action. Well at least we are talking about it. How scary is this? Our children our developing adult disease, and obesity is behind the wheel.

Osteoarthritis

Osteoarthritis, which affects the muscular/skeletal system, is another disease that progresses much less slowly in a person who is maintaining a healthy weight. Let's clarify the difference between osteoarthritis and rheumatoid arthritis. The latter is an inherited autoimmune disease where the joints become extremely painful, and some patients are unable to use these joints at all when they are end-stage. Fortunately, today, many treatments and medicines are available to slow the progression and decrease the intensity of pain associated with RA.

Osteoarthritis is basically wear and tear of the cartilage and is often associated with age and obesity. Although a 170-pound man may develop arthritis when he's in his sixties or seventies, an overweight thirty-five-year-old man may get it much sooner. The pain can sometimes be unbearable, depending on which joints are involved—the knees especially can be quite painful. Some patients end up with the complete loss of cartilage and require knee surgery, but are not candidates for surgery because of the risks associated with going under anesthesia at such a high weight. Obesity, again, is a risk factor when undergoing surgery.

Breast Cancer

As scary as it is for every woman to consider, breast cancer is even more common among those who are obese. The reason is thought to be an increased exposure to estrogen due to the circulation of estrogen in adipose, or fat, tissue. For this reason alone, I often drag my butt out the door for a run when I'm in a slump.

Be aware that not all women who get breast cancer are overweight; it is just one of the factors shown to increase risk. So please, no matter your weight, always get your yearly mammogram.

Maintaining a healthy weight can help you look good and feel good, but remember, it can also lengthen your life span and improve the quality of your life.

Chapter Summary

Being overweight or obese can affect all of your body systems, leading to disease and health problems.

- The most common diseases associated with obesity are heart disease(s), diabetes, osteoarthritis, and breast cancer.

- Losing weight will lower your risk of developing obesity-related diseases.

Chapter 3

Could It Be My Thyroid? I'm Really Hoping!

I know what you're thinking: *I'm sure it's my thyroid. It has to be. I am eating the same food I always have, and exercising as I always have, and I just can't seem to lose weight.* Worse, I can't stop gaining. Unfortunately, the thyroid excuse is only slightly more realistic than the "I'm not fat—I'm big boned" excuse.

Now that you have some background about calorie counting and the dangers of obesity, let me give you some information about thyroid function. I myself prayed that I would have a thyroid condition, so I could blame my inability to lose weight on my thyroid. This is a question I get asked over and over again, and although low thyroid function is not an entirely uncommon medical condition, weight gain or the inability to lose weight is usually not due to a malfunctioning thyroid.

Truthfully, while thyroid disease and other systemic illnesses (medical problems) can cause weight gain or trouble losing weight, other symptoms are usually present as well. Particularly in hypothyroidism (low thyroid function), other symptoms include dry skin, hair loss, and constipation. (Constipation, by the way, involves more than one hard stool. Everyone has a clogged-up day now and again, but constipation means not having had a bowel movement in several days.)

For thyroid-disease diagnosis, I examine lab results in addition to hearing patient symptoms. Occasionally I will start patients on a very low dose of thyroid replacement and follow their lab results, if I am suspicious that they have low thyroid function. The tests measure not only TSH, but also T3 and T4. These are actual hormones that circulate in the bloodstream, and their levels are worth following if you have started meds. I have on occasion started thyroid replacement even when lab work is normal, but the patient seems clinically as if he or she may have a low metabolism. Sometimes you cannot just treat the lab—you have to listen to symptoms. Baldness, tiredness, and intolerance to cold are common symptoms (along with, of course, the well-known symptom of weight gain).

When I do prescribe medication without seeing a problem in the lab work, it is worth mentioning that I follow the thyroid levels closely afterward, making sure I do not give more thyroid medicine than required. At their follow-up appointments, many happy patients report that after starting meds, all of a sudden they feel like exercising and are having less trouble losing weight.

One other important thing to mention about taking thyroid medication long-term is that it can increase the rate of osteoporosis. You should have your bone density checked initially, and then every several years to follow. If you have a family history of osteoporosis, you may want to get screened starting at forty years of age.

Other endocrine disorders can result in weight change; if you have problems losing weight even while counting calories and exercising, you may need to be screened for those.

One more note on thyroid disease: if your labs are normal, and you are still struggling with weight loss and other symptoms, it may be worth a recheck on lab work. I once had a patient who had all the symptoms of hypothyroidism, but her labs were normal. I recommended my usual weight-loss plan, and she was still symptomatic six months later. She did manage to lose some weight on my plan of action, but a recheck of lab work revealed low thyroid function. I started her on thyroid replacement, and she did great. If you think you may have another medical condition, ask your physician to recheck lab work at some point in your treatment. Talk to your doctor, and don't be afraid to ask questions. No one knows your body like you do.

For those newly diagnosed with hypothyroidism (low-functioning thyroid), I will order a thyroid ultrasound. Although thyroid cancer is rare, it is still something I think about when a patient is first diagnosed.

Even if your hypothyroidism has been confirmed, reaching the correct dosage of medication can take a few rounds of adjustments. Remember that your physician is on your side, and wants you to feel better. But he or she really doesn't want to answer fifteen phone messages in a week because your symptoms are still not controlled. Once patients are started on medicine, I will have them come in for a follow-up visit to check lab work and see how they are feeling. Most patients will start on a fairly low dose of Levoxyl or Synthroid. If the patient is still feeling badly, I will add some Cytomel. This is a bit of T4. Your thyroid produces mainly T3, but it also produces some T4. If you are not managed on your initial medicine, ask about Cytomel as an add-on medicine. I have found Cytomel to be very effective in getting patients feeling energetic again. Remember that your doctor wants to treat you, not just your lab work, so mention your continued symptoms in follow-up visits.

In addition to thyroid tests, if you have symptoms, don't forget to be tested annually for high blood sugar with a simple urine analysis, finger stick, or blood draw. There are many people who are unaware that there blood sugar is starting to increase as a result of weight gain. Most insurance plans will cover at least a urinalysis with the annual pap. If you are uninsured, include in your yearly budget a physical, a pap smear and mammogram (if you are a woman). For men included in your physical are, also the tests mentioned above with an added rectal exam that screens for prostate cancer, and colon cancer. You can shop around among your local physicians, hospitals, and outpatient facilities for the most affordable tests, physicals, and screenings. Or you can go to the nearest airport for a free xray, breast exam, and mention terrorists, and you will find yourself with a FREE colonoscopy as well!

An annual physical should not cost more than $200, though the lab work and mammogram may be extra. Is this really more than you would pay the vet to do a physical on your dog? You are worth it, damn it—get it done! Treat yourself to prevention, please, and have your TSH (thyroid stimulating hormone) checked yearly if you've always struggled with weight management.

Okay, so now that you've been diagnosed with a thyroid disorder (or not), you want to lose weight. Where do you start? You guessed correctly: educate yourself. Review chapter one and start mapping out your weight-loss journey—your eating plan. The next step on that journey is exercise.

Chapter Summary

Thyroid disease can affect your ability to lose weight; have your doctor check TSH, T3, and T4 to start the analysis.

- If you have hypothyroidism, your doctor will start you on the lowest dose possible then reevaluate in a few months. Additional meds can supplement thyroid medications.

- If you're taking thyroid medication long-term, you'll also want to be checked for bone density, starting at age forty.

Chapter 4

Exercise with a Purpose

Okay a lot of you reading, hate to exercise, and I get it. It's not fun for everyone, but I cannot emphasize enough the importance of exercise. Many people start a program In January and fade out by Valentines Day. They are not able to commit to the idea of exercise. So thinking about this issue it made me realize that we needed a fresh spin on exercise. It will be like coating your broccoli in cheese when you were a kid so you could choke it down, and then eventually broccoli does not taste so bad. Now some people still hate broccoli and there are always people who hate to sweat. Here's my fresh spin, the cheese on the broccoli if you will.

To exercise successfully, you have to **exercise with a purpose**. What does this mean?

Most people can answer the question "What is the purpose of exercise?" That's an easy answer: to get fit, stay in shape, look better, and feel better.

But why is exercise so hard for so many people? Those who dislike exercise find it difficult to maintain a routine when there is no end in sight. Sometimes, no one has given them clearly defined goals. "Okay, now go exercise and report back to me in a month." "Get your heart rate up, burn some calories, eat well, and get in shape."

A bit vague, don't you think? But I gave these instructions over and over, without realizing that a lot of people don't really know how to go about any of this. Getting in shape can be a daunting task for someone who is not used to exercise.

It was not until I was about forty that I started to struggle with staying in my routine. I was losing focus, and more and more often, I was making excuses instead of exercising. It dawned on me: "We need exercise goals. We need a reason to exercise." And so I entered my first marathon.

Finally, I had something to work toward. I was forced to make a schedule, set a routine, keep my eye on the prize, circle the date in the calendar, and tell my family, "These are my goals, and I need your help to be successful." It became fun to work out again. I got to experience the excitement of finishing my first marathon. My family did get behind me, and my husband and kids helped out, allowing me time to train.

Sometimes, all it takes to get in shape is to explain to your family how important exercise is, and how much you want to reach a goal. But life often doesn't work that way, in which case you will need to find a purpose for your exercise. You and your family are more likely to accept the exercise routine required if you set goals. (I certainly need not have trained for an entire marathon, so don't get intimidated and throw this book away just yet.)

You can set reasonable goals that are suited to your fitness level. Maybe set your sights on a three-mile walk to raise money for your kids' school, or a tennis tournament. Get into a paddleboard group (big here in Florida, and really fun), or join a kickboxing group that may have competitions scheduled. After all, isn't this the way it worked when we were kids? We joined a soccer team, or practiced karate, with the goal of competing and winning our division. Games and goals keep kids excited about exercise, so why not use these principles ourselves as adults?

If you are not competitive, or hate being around people, then set personal goals, as I do. I don't hate people, but after a long week, the only company I want are my Beats headphones and my iPod.

Set a personal goal to complete a mini triathlon by the time you are thirty … or forty … or 80! Exercise with a purpose—it just makes sense.

My husband's great-grandfather never understood the need for exercise. He used to say, "If you leave a new car in the garage and never use it, it's still in brand-new condition when you take it out thirty years later." Difficult logic to argue with, especially when you're talking to an eighty-year-old man who is apparently still in fairly good shape (or, frankly, even still alive). So I never tried to argue that with him.

But as we all know, the benefit of exercise far exceeds the risk of getting a scratch on the paint, or losing a hubcap. In fact, you may lose some hubcaps, but you will feel and look much better. And when you are eighty, you will likely be able to carry on a lot of activities that an inactive person would not.

So, if you hate to exercise, or hate to sweat, I hope this gives you some encouragement. Find a goal, set it, and keep it. Give yourself a purpose—a reason to train.

Personally, my favorite way to exercise with a purpose is to combine my two passions: running and traveling. So I set a goal, pick a race held somewhere I have never been, run a 10K, half marathon, or full marathon, and then do some sightseeing! It is great, and you don't have to go far—the race can be within driving distance of your home. But races are also a great way to spend part of your vacation. Instead of coming home five pounds heavier, you may have lost, or for sure stayed even.

The truth is, exercise is not easy for everyone, and not everyone likes it. But it is a necessary part of managing a healthy body weight. It is the answer to so many problems that walk in my clinic. First and foremost, exercise helps prevent heart disease, and depression is high on that list as well. You can actually eat a lot more of the good-tasting food if you fill your prescription for "one pair of Nike tennis shoes" and exercise daily. (A colleague of mine actually wrote this prescription to a female patient. I think it may have pissed her off, as we never heard from her again.)

The point is, most people are looking for an easier answer. Exercise is not easy, and I find that spending a bit more time talking about how exercise can help, what kinds of exercise are available, when is a good time to exercise, and so on helps a lot of people think about how they can incorporate exercise into their daily schedule. It's part of my job to ask questions to get people thinking about exercise. I'll frequently ask these questions:

- Do you work? If so, what are your work hours?

- What type of work do you do—sitting, standing, a lot of physical work?

- What types of exercise have you tried in the past?

- What exercises do you like to do?

- Do you have access to a gym, or treadmill or stationary bike?

- Have you justified your inability to commit to exercise with millions of excuses?

Many of my patients get a glazed look in their eyes when I start asking these questions, and look like five-year-olds trying to escape some terrible punishment.

I have been lucky, as I have always craved exercise. I need it for stress management, and it has always been part of our family's regular routine. As a kid, I saw my dad run marathons. My mom also did some running and played tennis. (I guess you need stress relief when you have a house full of eight kids). In the winter, we'd ski as a family every weekend. Many people find that once they get involved in some form of exercise, they forget how they lived without it.

Exercise does something for your psyche that you can't imagine until you are in an exercise routine. You begin to set goals, which should be realistic; start with ten minutes a day for a walk or jog, and then, as you build up your tolerance, set the bar higher and continue to strive for new goals. I have found that setting goals keeps me interested in exercise.

Write down your goals for the next month, six months, and year. We are creatures who need structure and deadlines. If I tell patients, "Okay, you have to exercise," it's hard for them to see any structure or the proverbial light at the end of the tunnel. Without setting goals, I found myself struggling to exercise regularly.

When I ask my patients, "Do you exercise?" I never seem to get a definite no. I have heard responses like

- My job is very physical.//
- I have stairs in my house.
- I never seem to stop all day long.
- I am constantly moving.
- I walk my dog (does it stop to pooh, and smell all the pooh from other dogs?) (if so this is not really exercise)

Yes, all of these things are good for weight loss, but if you are not losing weight, it's not enough. I cannot stress enough the importance of daily exercise. I figure if I tell patients to exercise seven days a week, they will get in at least five, and that is probably adequate. Once you have arrived at your desired weight and you are continuing to exercise almost daily, you can actually eat what you want (in moderation, at least). What you'll probably notice is that with increased exercise, you will probably crave healthier food choices as well. Since you're putting more demands on your body, you'll actually crave more fruits and vegetables. Or you may just want more cake! So have an extra slice, if you are tracking your calories and you have had a good workout.

Once you start eating more healthfully, you will have even more energy for exercise. I know I sound as if I'm trying to hypnotize you into believing this is true, but it really is factual.

I had a patient once tell me with all honesty that she could not sweat, because she had an allergy to her own sweat. I realized my breath would be wasted trying to explain that this could not be physiologically possible, so I listened until she was finished with her excuse, and then proceeded to give her a prescription for a diet aid. I never saw her again; she may have died when the hot weather started, having had a fatal reaction to her own sweat.

I once asked a trainer, "Which exercise is the best for weight loss?" and he said "Running." Now, not everyone can run, but his point was that getting your heart rate up, sweating, and maintaining that exertion this is the key to a successful workout. Some other options include walking briskly, swimming, or using a stationary bike, recumbent bike, rowing machine, or elliptical glider.

Most workout machines today will track how many calories you've burned. Whether you are on a treadmill or an elliptical machine, the important information to keep track of is your time, caloric burn, and target heart rate. As you get older, your target heart rate decreases. This information is posted in every gym and on most equipment, or you can just look it up on the Internet.

You have to stop making excuses for not being able to exercise. This is your body and your life, and no one is going to make time for you other than you. The more you do now, the less you will hurt later. Keep your joints and heart and lungs moving!

Let me share with you my favorite calendar of excuses for why people are unable to exercise.

THE CALENDAR OF EXCUSES

January – It's too cold. When the weather warms up, I'll start exercising. (I have to point out that my medical practice is in Florida, not run out of a meat locker in Fargo.)

February – I just got back from Mardi Gras, and I promise I'm going to get in a routine for Lent. When the clocks change, I'll have more daylight. And then there will be no more king cakes needing to be bought and consumed.

March – It's spring break. The kids have been out of school, and it's messed up my schedule.

April – I think I'm in a rhythm. I have been working out three times a week. But Easter is coming up …

May – God, it is really starting to get hot out there, but I'm going at least twice a week.

June, July, and August – It's just too hot here in Florida to walk outside. Plus I'm on vacation, or I have company all summer.

September – The kids are back in school, and it's messed up my schedule.

October – The weather is so nice that I'm really finding my rhythm, but I have to help the kids eat the Halloween candy.

November – The holidays are here, and we're going away for the long weekend. I refuse to give any thought to calories during Thanksgiving.

December – The holidays are here, and we're going away, so I'll be out of town. I will really get going in January and set a routine for regular workouts.

You can always find a reason not to work out. You have to make exercise part of your schedule. If you travel, ask if the hotel has a gym. Exercise if you're at a family member's house. If you want to, you can make the time, and you will feel better than you ever have in your life. If you're at a family gathering, exercise is the perfect out: "I'm training for a race," or "My doctor has ordered me to get an hour a day." Just like that, you can escape for a short time!

Dysmenorrhea (excessive menstrual cramps), depression, anxiety, heart disease, stroke, high cholesterol, type 2 diabetes mellitus and type 1 diabetes mellitus, osteoporosis … these are just a few health conditions that can be prevented or at least partially treated with exercise. If all my patients exercised as I recommend, my schedule would be empty for days at a time. I cannot live without my exercise, which is either a slow jog or time on a stationary bike. If I miss too many days, I get very irritable and cannot sleep well.

Find exercise that you enjoy. This should not be a time of day that you dread, or you won't stick to it. For some, this may be horseback riding; for others, swimming. If you need to vary types of exercise, please do so. There are certainly days when I don't want to run, so I'll throw in a thirty-minute bike ride instead. Also, pick exercise that is realistic. If you don't have access to a pool, don't vow to swim every day. If you live in Fargo, North Dakota, outdoor exercise in the winter won't work for you.

Just so you're aware, weight-bearing exercise does not mean lifting weights. It means bearing your own weight. So if your instructions from your doctor involve weight-bearing exercise, you need to walk or jog daily.

Chapter Summary

Exercise with the purpose of completing goals, not just to lose weight.

You may be big-boned or have thyroid disease, but you still need exercise.

- Find exercise you enjoy (or can tolerate), and begin a routine. Start slow with baby steps if need be. Gradually increase what you're asking your body to do.

- The family unit needs exercise, and we need to set examples for our kids. Don't just remain a spectator on the sidelines of their games.

- Exercise just makes you feel damn good—just admit it and get going!

- Choose an exercise that you enjoy!

Part Two
AGE AND WEIGHT

Chapter 5

Infants, Kids, and Weight Management

Childhood obesity is a real problem in Western culture. Data from the Centers for Disease Control and Prevention, listed on CDC.gov, has suggested that 17 percent of kids are obese in this country—not just overweight, but obese. And with this scary statistic, we have seen a rise in type 2 diabetes, which was not even a disease thirty years ago. Childhood obesity leads to adult diseases. It's time we took some action in trying to fix the problem, but how?

This chapter is so important, because the habits we instill in our children will last a lifetime. If you want your children to suffer from the side effects of adult obesity, start them on an "eat all the potato chips and fast food that they want when they come home from school, while they watch the same *SpongeBob SquarePants* episode for the twentieth time" plan. But if you want them to have healthy habits as teens and adults, you need to help them develop healthy habits from toddlerhood.

It is important to be a good role model, as well as expecting them to make good choices about food and activity. If parents have a healthy diet, don't overeat, and exercise regularly, children will follow. They don't really have a choice at a young age; if you buy and cook healthy foods and eat regular portions, so too will they. How many fat Japanese kids are there? None in Japan, because they eat sushi and rice. What could be healthier? It's not my taste, but it is healthy. The poor Japanese Americans come over, adopt our diet, and end up with Western health problems.

Weight management for infants and young children can work. I should also address the problem of malnutrition, which is obviously not a common problem in Western society, as we don't see weekly articles on "How to get your child fatter by Christmas" or "Have your kids beefed up before school starts."

First of all, after kids switch to cow's milk at twelve months of age, they should be drinking whole milk, unless you have cleared another choice with their family doctor or pediatrician. Kids this age need a diet of approximately 30 percent fat for proper mental and physical development. You can check these numbers with your pediatrician, who can in turn refer you to literature supporting that approximate percentage. There is a lot of great information on the American Academy of Family Practice (AAFP) and the American Academy of Pediatrics (AAP) websites—aafp.org and aap.org, respectively.

Children's central nervous systems are still growing, and their brains are still developing pathways for mental and physical growth. Now is not the time to restrict their fat intake, unless they are already obese or have some other problem.

I have seen patients whose parents are so obsessed with being thin that they have switched their twelve-month-old child to skim milk. This is *not* recommended. Listen to your pediatrician, and follow the correct plan. I have seen infants and toddlers who are underweight and dehydrated due to lack of nutrition. Please feed your children a balanced diet right off the bat. Check with your local physician or pediatrician for advice, especially if you are not sure what a balanced diet entails. An infant's diet should include much more fat than ours, for starters, and their need for protein is higher than an adult's as well.

In addition to basic nutritional needs, let me also address the conflicts about food that occur between parents and their children. A lot of parents really struggle when their children won't eat anything but a handful of Lucky Charms—or, in my children's case, Goldfish and Lucky Charms! It then turns into a fight between the two parents, and can also put a real strain on a marriage. Usually one parent is stricter than the other, and that strict parent's philosophy seems to be that a child needs to eat what is on his or her plate—and if not, too bad. Then, you see Mom (usually the one to give in) slipping the child an ice-cream sandwich when Dad is not looking, so the child doesn't "starve to death in the night."

This sets up two major problems. First, parents are divided, and thus easier to conquer. The first rule in winning a battle, after all, is "Divide and conquer"! In order to avoid an ongoing war, parents must maintain a united front. Talk with each other and come up with some rules you are both comfortable with, so the kids are not confused. Kids can thrive on a struggle in the home regarding food, and take advantage of it.

Children can make their parents crazy, because they won't eat what is for dinner, and it becomes a battle of wills. Kids learn very early in life that the two things they can control are pooping and eating, and they use that power to drive their parents crazy. (Most of the time, kids don't know they can do this at first, but when they get hip to it, you are screwed.)

These conflicts are a phenomenon of kids being able to exert their control, and finding out that they are not an extension of Mom and Dad. Children will test their parents' boundaries, and if you don't provide a united front, everyone will get frustrated.

The second thing they learn quickly is that if they don't have a daily poop, it stresses out Mommy. You may try, but you can't poop for your two-year-old son. Regular BMs seem easy for girls at the toddler age, but boys will often hold their poop, and then, if they have a giant, swirly poo, it hurts—and they don't want to go ever again! Well, knowing this is not an option, you once again have to let it happen as it is going to. They will finally learn that if you don't care if they poop or not, they don't, either.

I have had parents bring their children in specifically for an inability to poop daily. Oh, well, as with eating, they will eat when they are hungry and poop when they can't hold it any longer. Please consult your physician about other possibilities, especially if weight loss or fever is associated. Also, get some help if the issue lasts more than two to four weeks.

So back to kids and eating. I do not advise parents to sit down and make their children eat what's on the plate until it is gone, to the point that the children are gagging or feeding the dog under the table. Maybe when you were a kid, you sat there until all the food was gone, and you had to be creative—store food in your cheeks and regurgitate it later into the toilet, or feed it to the dog, or wrap it up in a napkin and empty the contents in the disposal or outside. My parents wondered why raccoons hovered around our house all the time, looking for food! My other favorite technique was to spread food around the plate to make it look as if I had eaten more than I really had.

So what is the answer? Remember that not all kids respond to the same techniques. Do offer healthy fruits and vegetables on a daily basis, and eventually your children will start to eat them.

I have put broccoli on my fifteen-year-old's plate for twelve years, and he occasionally will eat it if there is enough butter or gravy on it. It takes time for their taste buds to develop, and their tastes are constantly changing. Think about the first time you had some food that made you gag that you now love. For me, that question brings back memories of eating oysters for the first time. I was born and raised in Canada; I could not tell you what an oyster was. The first time I met my in-laws, my mother-in-law made oyster po'boys, since my husband's family was from Louisiana.

First, what is a po'boy? Because it looks like a sub sandwich to me. I bit into what I thought was a sub and found myself eating some chewy, gritty, nasty, loogey-like substance that had been deep fried. Yikes! I almost vomited, but it was my first meeting with my husband's parents, and I knew that at some point he would be sitting at my Polish grandmother's table, eating headcheese and cabbage soup. So I swallowed and survived, and now I love oysters—even raw. Yum!

If kids realize the food and bathroom battles does not bother you anymore, they will drop it and eat when they are hungry and poop when they need to. Once again, I've been through both with my own kids. I have had one who would not poop, and one who would not eat. I had a patient who was a psychologist, and damn it if his kid would not poop, either. We had this kid on prunes and Metamucil, and still he would hold his poop for days.

The other concern I have is that parents are too hung up on their own appearance. All that can be found in the house is fat-free milk and tofu. Kids cannot grow healthy on this. They need much more fat than the average adult to perform at higher levels, especially if they are participating in sports.

Many children are undereaters, but the more concerning problem in this society is the overweight family, including the children. Food is and has the been the center of an overweight family system. It starts when parents use food as a manipulative tool. The kids are fussy, so we give them M&Ms. I am just as guilty. I, too, have several Coach bags with melted chocolate at the bottom, which I have kept as a "shut-up food."

It is okay to do this in an emergency (e.g., if your two-year-old is singing "Happy Birthday" at your colleague's mother's funeral—true story), but not at every turn. This is how we start our children's habit of eating for comfort. You don't want your children to learn that food is for comfort.

Childhood obesity is at an all-time high. We are diagnosing twelve-year-old kids with adult-onset diabetes, because they are over two hundred pounds. And it seems to be a problem isolated to this society. My son and I spent some time in Europe one summer, and he was shocked at how few fat people we saw. I also pointed out that we had seen very few super-skinny people. I asked him on the way home how many fat people on scooters(the kind used here in the US) we had seen he answer was "none"—we had seen plenty of people on motorized Vespa scooters, on regular bikes, and on foot. The elderly population even were biking, climbing stairs, and walking up steep slopes like mountain goats. My educated guess after an occular patdown of the Europeans, suggest they experience a lower incidence of obesity and therefore diabetes. I have no studies to refer to, but it is and has been evident to me that lifestyle is a major role player in weight management.

In addition to feeding your kids a good balance of foods, try to stick to some kind of exercise routine. It is important for children to develop the habit of exercising and to see you doing it for the benefit of your long-term health. If you exercise, and it is important to you, it will be for your children as well. When my dad ran marathons thirty years ago, it was considered crazy. My mom and brother used to jog along the county highway north of Toronto, and people thought they were running from something.

But now, the rest of us all exercise on a regular basis, and our children are learning that this must be an important part of their daily routine. Your kids need exercise! Families can set goals for exercise and fitness. My kids play soccer, basketball, and tennis at different times of the year, and they swim a lot in the summer. If they are not involved in a sport, they both initiate exercise at home by using the treadmill or doing sprint work outside. They occasionally work together, with my son helping to coach my daughter in soccer.

I can tell that they feel better after exercise. My nine-year-old has started running with me, and she can do two miles without stopping. She came home and told my husband, "Daddy, I have a runner's eye." She had asked me why she felt so good after a run, and I had told her it was a runner's high.

Kids as young as three can feel the psychological impact of exercise. Exercise should be discussed with your children on a regular basis. Please encourage them to be active in whatever they like. Carve out at least thirty minutes a day for physical activity for both you and your children. You can be creative. We like to play "driveway tennis"—no net needed, just rackets and a ball. You may have a more traditional approach, like a family walk every evening. God knows we can all do with at least sixty minutes less of television a day.

Case Study: Justin

I have seen far more obese children than underweight children. I had a child in my practice whose parents went through a divorce, and it was very difficult for this child. He started comfort eating at the age of six, and by the time he was a preteen, he was over two hundred pounds. Mom and Dad had made the mistake of literally "feeding" into his coping strategy; they let him eat whatever he wanted, because they felt guilty. In addition to this, both parents would comment about his weight every time he was in the room with me.

Here is the fastest way to alienate your child: talk about what you would like them to change. They will go in the opposite direction. After some counseling on comfort eating, and the long-term damage this child was suffering both psychologically and physically, we came to the decision that his parents were not allowed to talk to him about his weight, but they were to stop buying junk food and stop offering food as a reward. He started to lose weight and feel better about himself, and in turn, he taught his parents that they needed to head down a healthier path.

Since then, the entire family has gotten on the same page, incorporating exercise and a balanced, low-calorie diet. That child felt empowered, since he had been the one who initiated the changes. Lead by example, but also learn from your kids.

Chapter Summary

Establishing good eating habits early is the best strategy.

- Walk, run, or otherwise exercise with your children. If you exercise, so will they. Be the example!

- Use food as a reward very sparingly; it can set up a negative pattern for later life.

Chapter 6

Teens and Weight Management

Most people who have come into my office to discuss weight loss have struggled since they were kids. Starting in the teen years, so many factors play into weight gain, not the least of which is genetics. A lot of people who are fighting to control their weight have one or more obese parents. Teenagers are especially vulnerable to weight issues and often have extreme reactions to weight problems.

I wanted to make a couple of important points here. First, if you are a parent and your teen is overweight, do not tell your child that he or she is overweight. As a parent, the comments and actions you take may lay the groundwork for your kid's body image.

We all see that the more Mom and/or Dad harp on a problem, the more of a problem it becomes. The more parents push, the more children will retreat (and, in the case of food, eat even more sweets and other unhealthy snacks). There is a fine line between communicating with your teens and trying to control everything they eat. Once again, setting a good example by buying healthy foods and eating moderate portions is the best place to start. Don't be hesitant to address these issues with your family doctor.

Often this is the best way to initiate healthy communication between parents and children without starting a tug-of-war.

Those of you who follow college basketball may know the story of Dexter Pittman, a player for the Texas Longhorns. A young boy who struggled with weight and, more important, with self-esteem, signed with the Longhorns, and his hard work and courage allowed him to become one of the country's best basketball players, and likely a high draft pick for the NBA when he is ready. With the guidance of his family, coaches, and trainers, he has transformed his whole life. He now mentors other children who struggle with obesity. Your overweight teen may respond best to someone outside the family, especially someone who knows the struggles of being overweight. The point here is that it can be done. Obese children do not have to be obese adults. Helping your overweight teen may even involve outside counseling referred to you by your family doctor.

> **Case Study: Vanessa**
>
> In one family I saw, one of the kids really was overweight, and one of the parents continually reminded her that she was overweight and that she needed to change her choices and habits. The more the parent talked, the more weight this child gained. When they came in for a consult, I told the parents that they were not allowed to discuss diet with their teen—no talk of exercise, food, or dieting.
>
> I then told the young girl, "This is in your hands, and you have decisions to make regarding your weight and ultimate health." I empowered her to take control of her choices, and she started to exercise, make healthy choices, and lose weight. As Mom backed off, she was encouraged to do her own thing, and she gained control over her exercise and diet routine.

The other disturbing problem I have seen is how many parents will tell children that they are overweight or eat too much. Especially when said in the company of others, those statements can really negatively impact a child's self-esteem. Parents, be careful what you say to your kids. Be careful what you say about yourself or others regarding weight. These statements are where skewed body images begin, and where we start to see eating disorders begin. If you notice your child's weight going up and down, please consult someone—a family physician, a dietitian, or a nutritionist—for help.

Another factor in this growing problem is that many kids who were active as younger children are no longer involved in sports as teens. If they are not playing on a team or involved in sports, they *need* some form of exercise. It is much easier to continue these habits than to introduce them at the age of thirteen. Fire the yard man and make your kids mow the lawn (great exercise). Have them wash the windows of the whole house, inside and out. Let them take responsibility for washing the family cars. Many other household activities can get your kids' heart rate up and get them sweating.

The other encouraging statistic is that children and teens who play sports are less likely to get involved with drugs and other unhealthy choices. I'm not sure we really needed studies to prove this information. It's hard to smoke pot and be a great point guard, or even a good one. In fact, an athlete who smokes pot will probably forget to go to practice. If your teen is forgetting to go to practice, it may be time for a pee test.

If you are a teen reading this now, you are in an important time of your life. As soon as possible, start eating healthfully, controlling your daily caloric intake, and—perhaps most important—exercising daily. This exercise should be cardiovascular in nature, like biking, walking, running, or any type of aerobic exercise. There is so much to choose from, and you don't have to do the same thing every day.

Good luck to you parents who are struggling with teens. You can make a difference by setting a good example. Get help if you need it.

Chapter Summary

The teen years are already challenging; dealing with weight issues can make this time worse.

- Keep your teens active and give them opportunities to work up a sweat.

- Don't harp on exercise and food; just be a good example, and give them positive reinforcement.

Chapter 7

The Postpartum Weight Struggle

Every woman has at least one hilarious pregnancy story and over the years I have heard some funny stories. My favorite story is not related to weight, but it is just damn funny! When a good friend of mine had her first baby, she had been married only nine months, so both the relationship and family were new. She came home from the hospital with her new child after being filleted open like a catfish from her C-section. She was bleeding heavily (not from her wound), which is normal after childbirth, so she sent her husband upstairs to get some pads, since she was unable to walk up the stairs. He came back with two eye makeup-removal pads. When she told me this, I laughed so hard I had to hang up with her, because I was causing her stitches to split. We couldn't talk for a month without reminding each other of the story and laughing for at least thirty minutes.

Pregnancy has its entertaining moments, but some mothers aren't quite as amused by the weight issues that can come with it. I found myself in that category!

I remember the day after I delivered my first child, and my mom was helping me get up to the bathroom in the hospital. I got a glimpse of this large dimpled ass in the mirror, and because I had drugs on board, it took me a minute to realize it was own ass. My mom grabbed the sides of the gown, and pulled them together quickly covering the nightmare that was my butt. I started to cry, and said "I'm so fat Mom, its not just the pregnancy, because the baby is already out!" Her response as all good mothers would say, "its just fluid retention honey, that will be gone in a few days". Well it took 6 months to get close to my proper body mass, and made me realize how we can justify the amount of weight we carry.

For example, let's say it's your first pregnancy, and you go into delivery weighing forty pounds more than when you started. Then the labor-and-delivery nurse informs you that you have given birth to a healthy seven-pound baby. You're so happy, because the baby is healthy—plus, you figure the placenta must weigh close to thirty pounds, right? Wrong.

Okay, maybe you can attribute another ten pounds to fluid retention. You still have twenty to go, so you understand that you have an extra twenty pounds of too many cupcakes and French fries to make up for. Once you have accepted that you have some fat to lose, you can start to think about a weight-loss program.

This may be the first time you've had to struggle with weight management. It's easy to gain forty to fifty pounds during pregnancy; after all, you are eating for two. You figure that you're going to get fat anyway, so you throw caution to the wind and have that extra piece of cake. Remember, though, that if you're not hungry, you shouldn't eat—even when you're pregnant.

Those of you who had already started gaining weight in anticipation of conception may have gained a little more than the doctor-recommended 25 to 30 pounds. That was me. Finally, I had a chance to eat without discrimination! After I gained 50 pounds with the first pregnancy, I vowed that if I ever got pregnant again, I would stick to a 30-pound weight gain. All right, for those of you already laughing, you are right to laugh—the truth is that mothers experiencing a second pregnancy are much more likely to gain weight. I gained 70 pounds with the second one. I steamrolled into the delivery room at close to two hundred pounds in the last trimester, with the momentum of a freight train.

I had told my OB—who, by the way, was female—and she had told me not to worry too much. If I hit two hundred pounds, I would have to take us both out. In an attempt to justify my weight gain, I figured on 10 pounds for the baby, 5 pounds for placenta, 10 pounds for boobs (at least 4 pounds each, and boy, are those fun to carry around) and 50 pounds of fluid. Yes, 50 pounds of fluid—I carried a lot of "fluid." My sweet mom kept telling me, "It's just fluid, honey. It will come right off."

After the baby came, I lost 20 pounds in two weeks—only 50 to go. I figured that for at least three months, I could use the "I just had a baby" excuse to explain how fat I was. But into the fourth postpartum month, still holding steady at 173, with my thighs still closely acquainted with one another, I knew it was time to take action. So I put my weight-loss education to work. I counted my caloric intake for the day and then subtracted calories burned during exercise.

Don't be unrealistic in shedding those postpartum pounds. If you expect to get into your size-six jeans two weeks after the baby comes, you may realize that sleeping becomes more of a priority than weight loss. Here is a tip, though: do get rid of all maternity clothes by three months postpartum. It's not good for your psyche to be wearing these for too long. I know they are comfortable, but you may be deceived into thinking you have lost more weight than you actually have.

Your caloric requirement will be increased if you are nursing. One of the many benefits of breastfeeding is an increase in metabolism, which helps you burn more calories each day. You may require up to 2,000 calories a day; be sure to check with your OB on this topic. I was not Mother Earth myself; I could not wait to strap these pregnancy porno boobs down with an ice pack and get back to running and a normal life. "For recreation only" was my motto about my breasts. Breastfeeding is great if you can do it and aren't working crazy hours, as I always have, and if you are comfortable doing it, but it's not for everyone. Don't let the lactation nurses tell you otherwise. Once again, educate yourself and make an informed decision on which is best for you and your family.

Again, breastfeeding does not give you an excuse to eat indiscriminately. You may actually find that you have to watch your diet if your baby has colic or seems to have an irritable GI tract. Understand that as your hormones are erratic and changing, your craving for certain foods can become strong, just like in pregnancy. That is okay. Just make sure to count calories, and try to stick to your allotted calories for the day.

Postpartum depression can also play a role in weight loss—or the lack thereof. I had bad postpartum depression after my first baby. I did not realize that it was a problem for weeks. Prior to having my second child, I started on antidepressants, and it helped tremendously. Depression can lead to overeating, just as it can lead to undereating. Ask your doctor if depression seems to linger for more than a week postpartum.

At my newborn exams, I always ask the mother how she is doing, and very often, the mother will tear up and admit that she's having a rough time. You are not a bad mother because you are depressed. It's bad enough that you are no longer the center of attention, but now you are fat, the baby is cute, and you're tired and feeling ugly. To top it off, if you have a girl, she's prettier than you, even without hair. You may think, *I can't stay fat and ugly. No one will ever believe this is my child.*

In fact, an acquaintance of mine told me after I had my child, "Your daughter is so beautiful. She looks nothing like you."

Thanks. Next time, just kick me in the gut. It's simpler for both of us.

No matter what our babies looks like, they look like us. We did the work, and our daughters look like us, damn it! And really, ladies, the race is on. You *can* get to a somewhat lower weight and look as pretty as your new baby girl in all her awesome outfits.

In the meantime, you have one pair of fat jeans, one pair of casual pants, and maybe something big and black in case someone dies. You are stuck in a wardrobe nightmare. Good luck if you have to go back to work. I was lucky; scrubs are awesome. Even if you're fat, they are always comfortable, but they can lull you into forgetting that your clothes do not fit.

For weight management, first I'm going to tell you to chill out until the baby is sleeping through the night. Do not try to get out there and run five miles when you have slept a collective five hours in two nights. I gave myself a few months to not worry about how I was going to come from 170 back down to my pre-pregnancy weight of 120. You cannot be concerned about your weight until you have been sleeping and have the energy to get back in the swing of fitness.

If your husband mentions your extra weight, remind him that you can lose weight, but he can't stop losing his hair. Men, please don't tell your wife she is overweight or needs to drop a few pounds. Believe me, she is well aware! The only words that should be coming out of your mouth should be words of encouragement. Your wife is tired, overweight, and maybe depressed—she needs words of encouragement.

Now, you may see a new mommy who looked as if she swallowed a small rodent instead of a basketball, and who snaps right back post delivery. A few weeks later, she's wearing the jeans she's had since her freshman year in high school and a midriff tee with her bellybutton showing. Try not to compare. You can always find someone skinnier, or someone fatter. Compare yourself to the fatter woman if it makes you feel better, but generally it's best not to compare at all.

Just work on you, and where you would like to be. Think about your target weight, and consult your doctor for some guidance. Set realistic goals for where you would like to be at three months, six months, and a year. For many, ten pounds in two months (meaning beyond the actual baby loss) is realistic. Thirty pounds in six months is doable as well. Human beings naturally enjoy structure, and setting goals helps us focus on where we want to get to.

So now that you've given yourself a break for putting on a few pounds after having a baby, take time to make a fitness schedule. You are already concerned about the feeding, sleeping, and pooping schedule, so give fitness some time.

As a corollary, you can't blame your weight on having had children. After three months, it's probably time to work your way out of your maternity pants and toward a more reasonable weight. Pick a target weight and get logging your caloric intake.

Most important at this stage is getting back into the swing of some kind of exercise routine. Not only will exercise boost your mood with endorphins, but it will also give you some alone time. This is important. Let everyone in your support team and family know that you need thirty to sixty minutes of alone time. You will love it and look forward to this time of day—even if, once in a while, you walk around the corner and sit down with a Diet Coke. Once you feel as if you're able to get some cardio two to three times a week, start tracking your weight and intake to see where you are.

Go into pregnancy with the knowledge that you are likely to gain weight, and that you will be determined to get back into shape after pregnancy. During pregnancy, it's a good idea to continue your regular exercise routine, after consulting your doctor, so that when the baby comes, you'll have less trouble getting back up and running.

You may have to change the type of exercise you do while you are pregnant. I have had several patients that are runners, and by four or five months, it's tough to keep running. Switching to walking, biking, or a mild aerobic class may be more comfortable. I switched to a stationary bike and found this to be very easy on my body, and I was able to keep this up until delivery. I know—how did I get so fat while still doing cardio three to four times a week? It's the intake, folks—lots of cake. Intake seemed to negate my exercise as far as calories burned, but my cardiovascular system was still in good shape after my daughter was born. This really made it easier to get back to running, as my lungs and heart were still accustomed to regular exercise.

So find what works. Don't overeat during pregnancy, but if you do, that is okay, too. You can and will find a way to lose the weight and get back in shape.

Chapter Summary

You will gain weight during pregnancy. Accept it, live with it, and know that you can lose it later.

- Set realistic goals for weight loss after the birth. Until the baby is sleeping through the night, your focus should be on basic maintenance, like healthy eating and sleep. Weight loss can come later.

- Pushing a stroller is good exercise! Consider this as a true "baby step" toward weight management after pregnancy.

Chapter 8

Menopause and Weight Management

Many of you got through life with no problems with weight gain. Even after children, you seemed to have no trouble returning to your prepregnancy weight. But then menopause hit, and if you are reading this section, it is likely that you have gained ten to fifteen pounds around menopause. The average age of menopause is fifty, and almost every woman I have seen in my office at this stage has complained of at least ten pounds of extra weight. Why is this?

Here is my theory, based on what I've observed in my hundreds of patients over the years. We know that adipose (fat) tissue causes higher levels of estrogen to circulate in the bloodstream—hence the higher risk of breast cancer associated with obesity. As your ovaries lose the ability to produce estrogen, the extra weight circulates more estrogen, which is probably one of the body's defenses against osteoporosis.

One patient was well past fifty; she was the mother of seven and the grandmother of many. For several visits, she complained that she thought she looked overweight. She was around 150 pounds and five-foot-seven, and I always thought she looked healthy and young for her age. I mentioned to her that most women will gain some weight after menopause and asked her whether she had ever seen women on the beach who were older and too thin. She answered yes, and we laughed about how unattractive that can be.

Remember Magda from *There's Something about Mary*, who believed that you can't be too thin or too tan? You *can* be too thin and too tan—though I believe Magda was actually orange! I told my patient that no one wants a grandmother who is stick thin; it's not what grandmas are supposed to look like. So for all of you women out there who are carrying a little extra, it's okay. You look better, and your body is trying follow its natural course. Weight gain may not be a bad thing if you have always been extremely thin. Be comfortable in your own skin.

This doesn't mean it's okay to get complacent with weight gain. If you are not tracking your intake, you will gain a lot more than fifteen pounds, and it is really hard to get it off. Go into menopause knowing that five to ten pounds is okay, but stop there and see what your body requirements are to maintain your desired weight.

If you have gained more than ten to fifteen pounds, or you are just not comfortable, pick a target weight and get to work exercising and managing those calories. Once again, you'll be sticking to the same plan of intake and burn.

The one good thing about this age is that you probably have more time to exercise and take care of yourself. If your kids have flown the coop, you have more time. If you're retired, you have more time. You'll have no excuse for not exercising at this point. Even if you are still working, you should have more time to devote to your own health. Find a good time for exercise and set a goal of doing cardio four to five times a week. That exercise can differ, too. Many women will do spinning one day, and then the elliptical machine, and then cardio weight lifting, and then Jazzercise. Variety can help prevent boredom.

During and after menopause, make sure you are getting regular physicals and ask your doc about bone-density testing. I like to get a baseline somewhere around forty-five to fifty-five, depending on risk factors (being of Northern European descent, being tall and thin, taking thyroid medication long-term, family history, and so on). If your numbers are heading toward osteoporosis, talk with your doctor about which path is the best for you to help prevent further bone loss and, in some cases, to rebuild bone.

Hormone replacement remains a source of controversy, so talk to your doctor about this. Everyone has different risk factors, and some women can't live without hormone replacement. Estrogen is actually the first line of defense against losing bone density. Next, depending on your numbers from the bone density, bone-rebuilding medicines like Fosamax, Boniva, Actonel, and Reclast work great. I am a big believer in bone rebuilding due to the decreased quality in life I have seen when women break a hip or fracture a vertebrae in the spine. This can be so painful.

Now, many patients have voiced concerns about the bone-rebuilding meds I just mentioned. In my experience, women taking these medicines may have a mildly upset stomach or reflux. This decision should be made between you and your doctor. Can we guarantee you won't have untoward side effects? Of course not, but many physicians won't prescribe estrogen or Fosamax-like meds for the fear of getting sued. Unfortunately, this fear plays an all-too-important role in many decisions we physicians make. I try to treat my patients as if they are family members. What would I tell my mom or sister? Then I try to educate patients, recommending that they do a lot of reading and their own research, so we can then decide together.

The bottom line is that if you are going to worry every day that you are going to lose bone in your jaw or get breast cancer from estrogen replacement, please don't take it; it is not worth the daily worry. Being consumed with concern can be as damaging to your health as other risk factors. I really believe that excessive worry leads to many health issues, such as binging and comfort eating.

Remember that after menopause, you are likely to gain ten to fifteen pounds, and of course it goes right to the tummy. "Where is my waist?" you might find yourself asking. "Yikes!" Well, this is the natural course the body takes, but this does not mean you can't keep a great body shape and eat healthfully. Such weight gain is very frustrating, and sometimes all it takes is for women to tell me how frustrated they are with weight gain and their changing body shape. A quick explanation on the natural course of the female body changes during menopause can help many women become less frustrated and focus on a healthy body weight, eating healthfully, and tracking calories, adjusting caloric intake as needed.

It is interesting that when people age, they gain weight, and then they seem to lose it as they approach seventy. I suppose it is a huge caloric burn to just keep the body alive past a certain age. Think about how many fat eighty-year-old people you have seen. Not too many! They have either had a heart attack from being too fat, or their metabolism has changed, and now they can eat whatever they want without gaining weight. So take solace knowing that if you make it to eighty, you won't have to worry as much about your intake—and frankly, you probably really won't give a damn. And guess what? You shouldn't. Enjoy ice cream, Christmas cookies, and birthday cake—even when it is no one's birthday.

Chapter Summary

Postmenopausal women will almost always naturally gain ten to fifteen pounds; this is normal. If it's too much for you, make a plan to lose it.

- Hormone-replacement therapy can help with weight management. Discuss the risks and benefits with your doctor.

- Bone loss is also a significant health risk after menopause. Up your intake of calcium and vitamin D, and discuss supplements with your doctor.

Chapter 9

Men and Weight Management

Since you men have lost your exclusivity privilege at Augusta National Golf Club, I felt bad and thought I would include a chapter just for you. This may be the only thing left just for men.

Initially, I thought this chapter would be really short. How to help motivate men lose weight? Perhaps a Hooters poster placed strategically in your man cave will remind you of the girls you want to date. Many men are motivated by sex, so I thought I should just include is a life-size poster of a *Sports Illustrated* swimsuit model. Hang poster, work out, get girl. Chapter over!

But having been married for twenty-one years, I most definitely do not want my husband to have a *Sports Illustrated* poster—I don't need reminders that I will never look great without airbrushing. Then I consulted my brother, who is closing in on fifty, and he gave me advice about men and managing weight. In this chapter, I've included information gathered from my brother in addition to wisdom gained from helping male patients lose weight over the last fourteen years as well.

These days, men are just as concerned about their appearance as women, if not more concerned. Does the term *metrosexual* ring a bell? A few years ago, the word was new to me, but I've since found out what this really means. When I heard this term for the first time, I was very confused. I learned from some younger women that it refers to men who are well-groomed (both upstairs and downstairs—also known as manscaping) and have more shoes than I do—and not just any shoes, but Cole Haan leather shoes. Shoes for every event. My husband had one pair of shoes when we were dating: tennis shoes. What a nightmare when we had to attend a wedding, funeral, or other formal event.

The point is that men are as vain as women. They want to be fit and manage their weight as well. They want to look good!

How is weight management different for men than women? Mostly, men have a different metabolism. Lucky for them, they seem to be able to lose weight more easily in their thirties and forties. Ladies, if you have ever considered having a contest with your spouse or boyfriend to see who can lose weight the fastest, forget it. They can lose five pounds in a day. I'm not sure why, its one of those questions I cant answer.

For men older than forty, losing weight is not so easy. At this age, many men typically are sitting at a desk and helping with the kids, having no time to get to the gym. It is as important for men as it is for women to find that thirty to sixty minutes a day for exercise. Ideally, working as a team is helpful for both. Trade off time, even if that means that you each only work out every other day. It's better than nothing, and your kids will see how important this is and learn that exercise is just another part of the day.

Men can manage their weight in much the same way women can: by monitoring calories in and calories out. But I wanted to also mention testosterone and its role in weight management. Like many women who enter the fabulous stage of menopause and experience a decrease in estrogen production, men can also experience health issues from reduced testosterone, including the inability to lose weight. If you notice that you are struggling with weight loss, and are exercising and eating well, consult your doctor to check your testosterone level. Treatment can help you muster the energy to get back out there to the gym. It also will help your body with other symptoms, if you know what I mean. That's right—it comes down to sex again.

I wanted to mention eating disorders as well. I am seeing male teens with eating disorders much more often than I used to early in my practice. Is it the skinny-jean phenomenon? I don't know, but as mentioned, men and women are equally concerned about their appearance. They also feel pressure to make weight because they wrestle or play other sports that require weighing in prior to competition. Being involved in sports is a great way to keep weight under control and maintain physical and mental health, but sometimes things can go too far. Although obesity far outweighs anorexia, keep an eye on your teen boys at home, and really be aware of their eating habits.

As mentioned, I enlisted my brother for help in the difference between men and women and weight. His insight informed me that men really love to eat. More so than women, men love to eat. Who has the largest pile of food on his plate at Thanksgiving? My father-in-law. Guess what, men? You are no longer hunting and gathering. You are just eating, and that lack of a caloric burn means trouble as you hit middle age. My brother is also a culprit of eating until he is ill—and then eating more.

My sister-in-law called me once to tell me that my brother had overeaten and thrown up, and thirty minutes later was hungry and went back for more. He is a guy who loves food, and anyone who loves food needs to exercise. There is no other option. Do more push-ups and more push-aways (push away from the table).

Most men who are sitting at a desk and getting no exercise require an average of 1,600 calories a day. As you add exercise, that number may go up to 1,800 a day. These numbers are an average—so count calories, be accurate, and determine what works best for you individually.

Men may have an easier time losing weight compared to women, but keeping it off is the struggle for all of us. Many men do have physical jobs, which helps burn calories, but understand this: just because you are on your feet all day does not mean you do not require exercise. When I mention adding exercise to a daily routine, I see a dazed look on male faces in return." But if you consistently exercise on top of the exercise you get at work, , you will lose weight and reach an ideal body weight". That message just does not get received when the patient is not ready to accept that they are either obese or well on their way to obesity.

As far as obesity-related health issues are concerned, men tend to develop heart disease at a much younger age than women, as well as high cholesterol and high blood pressure. Family history is also very important to men's health. Men who have dads, grandfathers, uncles, or brothers who have suffered heart attacks are at a greater risk themselves. Don't ignore chest pain, shortness of breath, or any other symptoms that are new or different. Consult a doctor and listen to your wife or girlfriend when they tell you, "That's not normal."

The men who really need to pay attention are those who are fit or look fit. Realize that you need to see a doctor if anything is not normal. Ask for that EKG or treadmill stress test that will screen you for heart disease. More information about heart attacks and strokes is available today than ever. You can read more about this topic at the American Heart Association's website, heart.org.

So, men, you have much more incentive to stay fit than just looking good! Make sure that when you consult your physician, you give a good family history and get the necessary screening, including cholesterol check, EKG if warranted, and a yearly prostate check starting at age forty. Screening for diabetes, heart disease, and colon cancer may be recommended. Many physicians will avoid telling patients to get yearly rectals, and I understand why. It's not the most glamorous part of my job, and not something men care to do on a yearly basis. However it is recommended yearly with the blood test screening for PSA (prostate-specific antigen).

Believe me, prevention is often the key to good quality of life. In addition to regular exercise, a yearly visit to the doctor's office is a must. Please don't show up at your doctor's office at age fifty-five, struggling with the tire around your middle and in need of weight-loss consultation. And then be surprised that you have diabetes and high cholesterol.

And if a big poster of a swimsuit model, helps, well … you're the one who will have to deal with your wife, not me! You may be lucky enough to have a man cave in your home where you can keep such items.

Case Study: Taylor

A patient of about forty-eight came to see me out of frustration with his spare-tire belly. He had tried exercise and the no-carb diet, but with no success. Time for a family history and physical exam.

He was not overweight by more that twenty pounds, but I came to find out that his blood pressure was elevated: 150/100 while in my office. Way too high!

He wanted diet meds, and that was all he was there for. So I started to ask about any new symptoms, his family history, his eating routine and his "exercise" (he had tried joining the gym, and he had been a spectator of college football since the age of eight, so in his mind, he was involved in exercising).

The first time he tried the treadmill at the gym, his belly bounced up and down, and he was next to the Hooters waitress who was outrunning him like a bloody cheetah on the next treadmill. So he got discouraged and came to see me for diet aids. Sound familiar?

We had to start to get his blood pressure down before doing anything else, and I let him know that if he lost twenty to thirty pounds, he may not need blood-pressure meds. That motivated him, as a lot of patients don't want to admit that they take any medication. So after his first visit, he got my spiel on exercise calorie counting—prevention!

He returned four weeks later a few pounds lighter and feeling better about himself. We checked his testosterone level as well doing as a lot of other blood work, and he was found to be in need of a testosterone supplement. We got him going again—moving, exercising, and tracking his intake. He actually did not require any diet pills and now comes to see me every six months to recheck his blood pressure, weight, and so forth.

What a great success story!

Chapter Summary

- Whatever motivates you for weight management is good. If that's sex, then fine. Looking good for the ladies is often a good motivator for maintaining a good body weight.

- Portion size and alcohol intake are both factors in weight management for men.

- In addition to weight management, baseline testing for various diseases are in order, starting at age forty, to maintain good health.

PART THREE

MOTIVATE THYSELF

CHAPTER 10

Supplements and Diet Aids

If you who skipped the rest of the book and started here, go back to the first chapter. There is no magic pill that will keep weight off forever. Remember NO MAGIC REQUIRED!

There are, however, some diet aids that I have used successfully with my patients. The one I use most is Phentermine, and I have also used Tennuate. Both have proven to be safe, and effective for the short term. Think as these as starters to get you going. They can also be effective for those who reach a plateau and can't get past a certain weight. They are by no means the answer to long-term weight management. When I start patients on this type of medicine, I monitor them closely to check their blood pressure and weight, and have them seen monthly in the office while they are taking medicine.

Some women find that these can be more effective used not daily, but on days when they may be more likely to fall off the wagon—like the annual holiday party or certain dates in their monthly cycle. Ask your doctor about a diet aid if you are already exercising, watching your intake, and tracking calories, and are still unable to get to your target weight. Not all physicians are comfortable prescribing them (and that is okay!), so you may have to see another doctor for weight management.

Okay, what about over-the-counter (OTC) weight or diet supplements or alternative, holistic remedies? Personally, I have not been trained in alternative medicine so I don't feel comfortable giving advice. Many physicians have training in this area, and they may have some helpful (and hopefully educated) advice.

As far as OTC aids, be careful, as a lot of them have not been researched, and not all are FDA approved. I have seen some patients suffer untoward side effects—mainly increased heart rate and blood pressure. But mostly these patients are not doing the most important part of weight management, which is exercising and counting calories. Remember that a lot of OTC supplements often include diuretics and stimulants that most people are unaware of. Sometimes these can result in long-term problems, such as heart failure. So avoid anything that isn't tested and approved; it is much safer to use prescription diet meds under the care of your doctor. Please don't order anything over the Internet—you don't know what is in it or where it came from.

Chapter 11

Odds and Not-So-Fat Ends

If you have gotten this far, you probably are serious about changing the way you look at food and weight management, and your overall health. Here are some tips that help me manage my own weight, and help my own patients as well.

- Remember that low-fat or low-carbohydrate foods can have just as many calories as the burger you were going to choose. Calories matter.

- Remember that raisins, grapes, and nuts are really high in calories. So are a lot of fruit juices. Read the labels, and get familiar with where calories are coming from in your diet.

- If you feel hungry, sometimes you're just thirsty; drink some water first. If you're not hungry, don't eat.

- A great low-calorie snack when you want something sweet

are sugar-free popsicles—only 15 calories per popsicle. (Don't eat the whole box. One or two is good.)

- If you're heading to a feast such as Thanksgiving dinner, get exercise ahead of time. Be honest with yourself: there is no way you are going for a run after five pounds of turkey, gravy, and stuffing!

- Throw out the calendar of excuses and write your own exercise calendar for weight management.

- Sign up for a local 3K or 5K as a long-term goal. It could start out as a short distance and then possibly a mini triathlon or marathon. Remember this: Oprah ran a marathon! You can, too, eventually. You can start out by walking, jogging, or biking for twenty to sixty minutes a day. Make time for yourself, and let your family know you are not available during that hour!

- Instead of coming home after work and having an alcoholic beverage to unwind, go out for a walk. This is a much healthier way to decompress. Instead of consuming 200 to 400 calories with just alcohol, exercise for 20 to 30 minutes and burn 100 calories –200 calories. Now you are at least 300 calories ahead for the day.

By following the tips above and implementing the concepts in the previous chapters, you can start your journey to weight management—and arrive at your destination!

Conclusion

A Patient Success Story

CB

Food an addiction? I am not addicted to food. People are addicted to drugs, cigarettes, alcohol. Not food. Who was I kidding? I loved food, I was addicted to food, I was an emotional eater, loved social gatherings because of food, and would eat beyond the point of being full. It was a sickness I had and had in common with thousands of Americans.

My wake up call was a day in 2011, when I went out with a group of people to celebrate a friend's birthday. We ate, danced, socialized, and had a good time. I thought I looked great getting ready to head out for the night. Matter of fact you know days you feel extra good? That was one of those nights. March of 2012 I was looking at the pictures taken from just that night and that was all it took. My face was huge, I looked swollen, I was the biggest one there, what I was wearing in fact didn't look that great, and I was FAT! It was a horrible reality check, but indeed one I needed. It lit the fire under my butt! I didn't want to be the "fat girl". I didn't want to be the one anymore that felt uncomfortable walking in a room. I didn't want to be unhealthy anymore. I didn't want to live my life for food anymore. I didn't want to shop in plus size clothing anymore. I didn't want to be tired all the time and have no energy anymore. I wanted to change, I wanted to make a lifestyle change, I wanted to be more active, and I wanted to look good, feel good, have self-confidence, and be comfortable in my own skin.

The very next day after seeing that photo I made the lifestyle change for the better in my life. At 220 pounds I didn't care what I had to do nothing was going to get in my way or stop me. I got rid of everything in my house that was not good for my body. I drank lots of water, cut all bad carbs, all sugar, watch my calories, watched my fat, and I finally put my dusty treadmill to use. I watched literally everything I ate and only made and make healthy choices and make it a daily part of my life. I stay active. That is the key you have to stick with it and stay active! With my will power, the advice and support of Dr. Lisa Clark, the support of friends and family I stuck with it and the pounds fell off. It is now October 2012 and my last weight was 158! I feel great, have more energy, look like I took off years on myself, and have self-confidence out of this world. People notice the change and it feels amazing. I feel like a whole new person, I am a whole new person. I will continue to live a healthy lifestyle and to better myself. Once your mind is there 100% you can do it. I am living proof and if I can do it anyone can do it and trust me it is worth every minute of it! Food was my addiction and I defeated it.

CB is a patient of mine who I have watched finally take her health and weight into her own hands. That is what this book is about. Understanding that losing weight IS NOT EASY. Keeping weight off is even harder. By education I hope I can motivate one person at a time to take responsibility and pass on their success to motivate others. I have witnessed other patients ask CB, what her secret has been for losing weight. And her response "there is no secret."

It's A Wrap

The average weight and body mass index continue to climb in this country. It is time to take control of what we are putting in our mouths and time to get some exercise. If we start, our kids will start, and hopefully we can stop this epidemic of obese children who then become obese adults. No one wants to be fat; most people just don't know what to do. I hope this short handbook has offered some motivation and some knowledge to those of you who have struggled.

In visits to my private practice, weight management comes up over and over again. Please don't be afraid to talk to your doctor about this or even ask to see a dietitian. Make sure your physician knows what your appointment is for, so you don't get a ten-second visit on weight after discussing something else for twenty minutes. It is often good to devote an entire appointment to weight management.

Remember that you have control over what types of food are in the home, and this can form good habits that will likely last a lifetime.

I wish for all of you a healthy life and a comfortable weight where you feel good in your own skin. Continue to exercise regularly. It will help you deal with the stresses of today's world.

I hope to take part of the profits from this book aid in education and action toward prevention of childhood obesity, and therefore adult obesity.

Good luck, and Bon Chance !'
Lisa Clark, MD

About the Author

My quest to become a physician began at the age of thirteen. While I wavered here and there in the process, I was able realize my dream of practicing medicine on the beach. I met several physicians along the way who inspired me to continue pursuing a career in medicine. A female friend of our family helped me realize that women could achieve success in medicine. She was a role model I thought of often along my journey.

I began studying premed at the University of McGill before meeting my husband and transferring to Louisiana, where I resumed studies at Southeastern University. I received a Masters degree at Southeastern Louisiana University. In 1992 I was asked to join the class of 1996 at Louisiana State University New Orleans, after being on the waiting list for 4 months. (continue to pursue your dreams). I graduated from Louisiana State University in New Orleans on time, in the summer of 1996. Subsequently, I spent three years as a resident at Tallahassee Memorial Medical Center, the last year of which I was co–chief resident.

I had my son, Adam, after my intern year, and I managed to juggle him between family and friends until I got out of residency. I set up shop with Twin Cities Hospital in Destin, Florida, near the beautiful beaches of the panhandle. I have maintained solo practice since, juggling work and kids. I had my daughter in 2003 and continued to work hours conducive to family life.

I love what I do. It is especially gratifying helping those who have struggled with weight and watching them make it to a place where they are comfortable. Thank you for inspiring me, to get this done. Please continue to inspire me, and inspire those around you, and for Gods sake LIGHTEN UP AMERICA!

Notes

Notes

Notes

Notes

Notes

Notes

Notes

Notes

Notes

CPSIA information can be obtained
at www.ICGtesting.com
Printed in the USA
FFOW02n1944240217
32819FF